HEALING YOUR SKIN THROUGH NATURAL CARRIER OILS

MON CHERI DAVENPORT

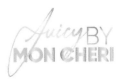

Book Design by HMDpublishing

CONTENTS

WHAT ARE CARRIER OILS?

C arrier oils are also known as base oils or fixed oils. They can be used to dilute essential oils. However, Carrier oils used along add powerful benefits and nutrients directly to your skin. Carrier oils are mainly sourced from the fatty parts of a plant, such as kernels, nuts or seeds. The Carrier oils covered in this book include Black seed oil, Olive oil, Grapeseed oil and Vitamin E oil.

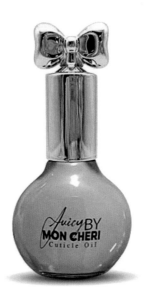

PERSONAL JOURNEY ABOUT HOW I GOT TO THE PLACE OF DESIRING TO TEACH PEOPLE ABOUT SKIN CARE AND HEALING

My journey to care about my cuticles and skin started when I was a youngster. I'm a nail biter and I have been biting nails for as long as I remember. I would bite my nails then move on to my cuticles until they would be very damaged, ripped and painful. That was my signal to Stop! The solution that was given to me was to use cuticle oil to help repair skin fast, by my mother, who was also a nail biter. So, I always had access to cuticle oil in my household and would regularly buy it as an adult. Fast forward to 2020 during the pandemic, when items bought regularly became distinct-ish. Cuticle oil was one of those things for me, which prompted me to solve this problem for myself. It allowed me time to think to myself, and create my ideal formula. Black seed oil is the number one ingredient on my list!

WHY BLACK SEED OIL?

So, in 2000 while still in college studying to be a Computer Engineer, I converted from Baptist Christian to Sunni Muslim. Becoming a Muslim opened me up to a new culture I was not accustomed to which included black seed oil. To become a Muslim you have to take the Shahada which states: There is no God but God (Allah – i.e. there is none worthy of worship but Allah), and Muhammad is the Messenger of Allah." It is the most sacred statement in Islam, and must be recited with full understanding and mindfulness of its meaning.

Therefore the statement.

Abu Hurayrah (ra) narrates that the Prophet (pbuh) said: "Hold on (use this seed regularly)! Because it is a remedy (cure) for every disease except death."

Abu Hurayrah (ra) narrates another hadith in which the Prophet (pbuh) said, "Allah (God) did not send down a disease without having sent down its cure."

Being told black seed oil heals every disease except death and because of easy availability of black seed products and black seed oil in most Halaal grocery stores, I eventually purchased some oil for myself to see the miracle on my own. I was a believer after those first cold symptoms one winter day. I made and drank some black seed peppermint tea. The result was prenominal, the next morning I was back to normal. I recovered faster than I ever remembered before. So, after that I used black seed oil at every opportunity possible to test its limits. I used it on rashes, open wounds, dry skin, hair growth, for myself, family and friends. Black seed oil is a staple in my family now. It stays in stock in the pantry as black seed seasoning and in medicine cabinets.

I breastfed all four of my children for at least 2 ½ years plus each. Whenever my nipples got to the point when they were raw and sore from breastfeeding, I would use black seed oil to soothe them as the oil is also healthy for baby to take. It's an easy way to give your baby black seed oil if they need it as well.

My two oldest children used to have eczema flair up often. Which I would successfully treat with applying black seed oil after cleaning them in the shower or bath. I used it on any bug bites and rashes on my children as well. And it always seemed to speed up the healing process. It helps to know I have a tool to use for most ailments for my facility without getting a diagnosis right away, so we can start the healing process immediately.

The reason black seed oil heals most things is because it is packed with nutrients and healing chemical compounds. The black seed has over 100 chemical compounds and nutrients. The nutrients, proteins and compounds have the ability to give your body nutrition that your body's system needs to balance and get to the natural health state. Our bodies know how to balance itself when it's given what it needs or lacks and knows how to use it.

So especially if someone is ill and doesn't know why, I would definitely recommend adding black seed oil into their diet via internally or topically as the skin has the ability to absorb nutrients. It could only help. I am a black seed super fan!

Therefore, I believe everyone should have access to black seed. I desire to add it to everyday products to help others heal naturally by getting nutrients they lack. It's the opposite of what the marketplace does. Currently, there are lots of everyday products that gives us toxic additives that help to deteriorate our healthy states. Black seed oil has the ability to counter this. This is the value that I will add to the world. Juicy by Mon Cheri cuticle oil and body oil is one of the first creations in this endeavor.

Since the creation of my incredible body oil recipe made with black seed oil, Olive oil and vitamin E oil plus proprietary essential oil blends, I have experienced better skin tone, a softer skin texture, fast healing scar repair and more. I have to show and share this with the world. I'm making it my mission to share it with YOU! Your skin will Thank you with incredible results.

My daughter has Psoriasis which is a skin disease that causes a rash with itchy, scaly patches, most commonly on the knees, elbows, trunk and scalp. Her neck has a darker tone, she gets rashes in her elbow pit, knee pit, and her scalp gets dandruff often. Now that she has used Juicy by Mon Cheri body oil formula, her skin tone, texture and dryness is improving daily. It's a WOW!

Let the Journey begin. I want to help you assess your skin type and then give you valuable information how to heal it naturally using natural oils available to us. I will provide you with small changes you can add to your daily routine to help you have Radiant skin for life simply.

Skin assessment

There are 5 major skin type categories. Though our skin can change throughout our lifetime, given different environmental scenarios. The skin types are Normal. Dry, Oily, Combination of Oily and dry and Sensitive.

Answer these questions below to help define your current skin type.

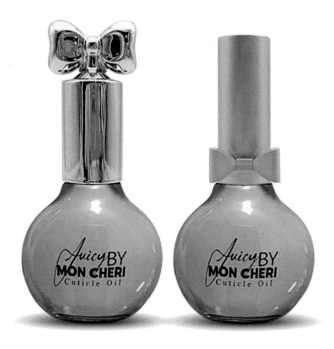

SKIN TYPE ASSESSMENT

The different types are: normal, oily, dry, combination, or sensitive skin types.

Which one do you have?

Your skin type can change from time to time. For example, hormones can affect your skin type during pregnancy.

What are the main factors that determine the differences? Factors include:

- How much water is in your skin, the skins elasticity level and comfort level
- How oily the skin is, which effects its softness
- How sensitive your skin is

It is important to determine your specific type to identify which skin care ingredients and products are optimal; it is equally important to understand which to avoid.

Normal Skin Type

Normal skin is neither too dry nor too oily. It has regular texture, no imperfections and a clean, soft appearance.

Normal skin can have:

- Few or no imperfections
- A glowing complexion
- Slightly visible pores

- No extreme sensitivity

Combination Skin Type

Your skin can be normal or dry in certain areas and oily in other areas which usually include nose, forehead, and chin. Lots of people have this type. Requiring different care in different areas.

Combination skin can have:

- Blackheads
- Shiny skin
- Pores that look larger than normal because they're more open

Dry Skin Type

Dry skin can crack, peel, or become itchy, irritated, or inflamed. If extremely dry, it can become rough and scaly, especially on the backs of your hands, arms, and legs.

Dry skin can crack leaving it more exposed to bacteria, although in general this is not serious, it may cause other skin disorders, such as eczema, or be more prone to infections if not properly managed.

Dry skin can have:

- Mostly invisible pores
- Dull, rough skin
- Red agitated patches
- Little skin elasticity
- Visible skin lines

Dry skin can be caused by:

- hormonal changes or ageing

- Medications
- Weather such as wind, sun, or cold
- Ultraviolet (UV) radiation from tanning beds
- Indoor heating
- Your genes
- Hot, long showers and baths
- Ingredients in cleansers, cosmetics, or soaps

Oily Skin Type

The oiliness of your skin can change throughout the changing seasons of year or the weather. Puberty or other hormonal imbalances like pregnancy, stress, heat or too much humidity also are culprits that can affect the oiliness of your skin.

Oily skin is caused by excessive fat production by sebaceous glands, and usually because of genetic and/or hormonal causes. Additionally, because excess sebum blocks pores and leads to acne, those with oily skin are prone to blemishes such as whiteheads and blackheads.

Oily skin can have:

- Blackheads, pimples, or other blemishes
- Shiny appearance
- Slick or greasy feel
- Visible or enlarged pores
- Makeup that won't adhere to skin

Sensitive Skin Type

Sensitive skin has triggers. You have to determine what they are to avoid them. There are a variety of reasons, however, often it's in response to skin care products applied to skin.

Sensitive skin is more prone to react to stimuli to which normal skin has no reaction. It is a fragile skin, usually accompanied by feelings of discomfort, such as heat, tightness, redness or itching. This type of skin loses its barrier (or protective) function, making it easy for microorganisms and irritant substances to enter it, and increasing the possibility of having an infection and allergic reactions. It is a delicate skin that needs more care to fight dryness, roughness and its usual appearance. Sometimes, it is referred to as irritated skin instead of sensitive, but these terms are synonymous and there are no dermatological differences between them.

Sensitive skin can have:

- Burning sensations
- Redness
- Itching and irritation
- Dryness

Mature skin

As the skin matures and ages, the body naturally slows production of collagen, sebum, hyaluronic acid and ceramides. These all serve to maintain skin barrier function, which improves skin elasticity and moisture levels.

Mature skin can have:

- Looseness
- Wrinkles
- dryness
- fragility

Additionally, mature skin often develops dark spots as a result of prolonged exposure to UV rays. Skin that has been exposed to significant amounts of UV radiation may experience signs of aging earlier.

HOW USING BLACK SEED OIL BENEFITS DIFFERENT SKIN TYPES

Black seed oil is obtained from the cold press of the seeds of the Nigella sativa (fennel flower) plant. This plant grows in parts of the Middle East, Asia, Eastern Europe, and North Africa. Black seeds are obtained from the plant of the ranunculus family (Ranunculaceae) grown for its pungent seeds, which are used as a spice and in herbal medicine.

It has been used for over 2000 years in Asian, Ayurvedic, and Arabic cultures for its medicinal properties. In ancient times people used it as a very good ointment (by mixing it with other herbs) for very severe wounds and infections.

The pure and natural black seed oil has a golden-brown color. It has a shelf life of 2 years and is non-comedogenic. Its scent can be described as mild, earthy, spicy, or woody. It is also referred to as black cumin seed oil, black caraway oil, black onion seed, or kalonji oil.

Black seed oil has equivalent beneficent if added to your diet. Black seed oil has thymoquinone, which is an antioxidant and anti-inflammatory, which helps in removing toxin chemicals and dust germs from your skin and provide you a brighter, smoother skin. They have a very good effect on the health of your skin. Black seed oil helps in reducing psoriasis plaques, acne symptoms, inflammation and bacteria in healing wounds. And improving skin moisture and hydration.

Black Seed Oil has an essential fatty acid profile made up of linoleic acid (50.2%), oleic acid (19.9%), and stearic acid (2.5%).

No matter what your skin type is, adding black seed oil to your skin will aid, heal, maintain and improve your skin.

- **Normal skin type**: The black seed oil has a high concentration of linoleic acid. That makes it capable of enhancing the absorption of other products into the skin. It goes a long way to render the other products in your skincare routine more effective as they will be able to reach deeper layers of the dermis.

- **Oily skin type**: Its linoleic acid content helps unclog pores and regulate sebum production in oily skin, while oleic acid provides hydration.

- **Dry skin type**: This oil equally works to smooth out signs of ageing. Its high concentrations of linoleic acid helps to boost ceramide production for a healthy lipid barrier.

- **Combination skin type**: This lightweight oil has antioxidant, anti-inflammatory, antibacterial, and antifungal properties that make it suitable for combination and acne-prone skin.

- **Sensitive skin type**: When exposed to free radicals, skin cells are damaged, causing inflammation in acne-prone skin. The antioxidants present in black seed oil help prevent that by reducing the oxidative stress and neutralizing free radicals present on the skin.

In Summary:

Dermatological scientific studies reveal that black cumin seed essential oil treats pathogenic yeast and dermatophytes fungi (a group of fungi that causes skin disorders). This includes skin conditions such as fungal acne, facial hair, and body ringworm, jock itch, onychomycosis and athlete's foot. These studies have shown black seed oil properties include antibacterial, antiviral, antifungal, antiparasitic, wound healing, anti-inflammatory (Psoriasis, Acne vulgaris), and treatment of skin pigmentation (darkening), hypersensitivity reactions (reduction), skin cancers and more. For these reasons Juicy By Mon Cheri oil products include black seed oil to achieve a naturally radiating skin head-to-toe for life.

HOW USING OLIVE OIL BENEFITS DIFFERENT SKIN TYPES

Olive oil is a nutrient-packed oil made from pressing olives and then expressing their oil. It is rich in healthy monounsaturated fats and antioxidants, which may benefit the skin when applied directly to it. Olive oil does have some reported benefits to the skin. According to the International Olive Council, olive oil has many vitamins, including A, D, and K, as well as vitamin E. Olive oil is also an antioxidant, so it might help prevent or reverse damage from cancer-causing ultraviolet radiation. It has a very high concentration of an ingredient called squalene as compared to the other types of fats and oils that humans normally eat. The squalene is what gives olive oil the extra antioxidant boost. It moisturizes and fights bacteria. If you're prone to acne, using a soap made with olive oil may help decrease your acne by killing off the bacteria that causes it. Olive oil is also known to moisturize and hydrate your skin. Olive oil is often used as an ingredient in face wash products. There are cosmetics that have olive oil bases. It can also be found in some soaps, body washes, and lotions. It's possible to use olive oil as a moisturizer without any added ingredients by applying it to your skin.

- **Normal skin type**: Moisturizes the skin. Known to be rich in healthy fats, olive oil is a great natural moisturizer that helps in sealing the moisture and forms a layer on the skin, which helps in protecting it.

- **Oily skin type:** It helps to regulate sebum production and prevents excessive oil on the skin. It also helps in giving you a supple and plump skin with its natural hydrating properties.

- **Dry skin type**: Olive oil acts as a natural moisturizer and helps in lending natural moisture. It is super easy to use olive oil. You can simply apply it directly on the skin. It exfoliates the skin. The antioxidants in olive oil helps in deep cleansing the skin and pores. It removes all the dead skin cells and gives fresh and radiant skin. Olive oil also helps in tackling acne marks and removes excess oil and dirt from the skin. Anti-Ageing. Dry skin is extremely prone to show early signs of ageing and hence olive oil is the perfect way to deal with it. It has excellent anti-ageing properties which helps in fighting fine lines, wrinkles and other signs of early ageing.

- **Combination skin type**: Olive oil is rich in antioxidants, which helps in fighting free radicals in combination skin type. It helps in retaining the elasticity of the skin and keeps the texture firm.

- **Sensitive skin type:** Cleansing the Skin. Deeply cleansed and glowing skin is like a dream come true. Olive oil helps in deeply removing all the dirt from the skin. It is rich in vitamin E and hence, is a great component for achieving clear skin.

Olive oil is an occlusive, which coats the skin and seals moisture inside so it doesn't evaporate. Olive oil is also an emollient, which means it smooths and softens skin, giving it the feeling of being supple and moisturized.

In Summary:

Olive oil moisturizes skin, reduces signs of aging, fights oxidative stress, increases collagen, cleanses skin, lowers risk of acne, promotes wound healing, has anti-inflammatory properties and prevents pressure ulcers. Therefore, the olive oil in the Juicy By Mon Cheri Body oils works well with the black seed oil and Vitamin E oil combination to achieve naturally glowing and radiating skin for life.

HOW USING GRAPE SEED OIL BENEFITS DIFFERENT SKIN TYPES

Grapeseed oil is a byproduct of winemaking. After wine is made by pressing grapes, tiny seeds are left behind. Grapeseed oil is then extracted from these leftover grape seeds using a cold-pressing extraction method. Grapeseed oil contains a natural store of antioxidants and skin-promoting compounds. High amounts of omega fatty acids, especially linoleic acid, and vitamin E help maintain healthy moisture levels in the skin. Phytochemicals like proanthocyanidins offer serious benefits for UV defense, as studies have linked these compounds to prevention of skin cancer. Grapeseed oil actually cures and manages acne breakouts, lightens acne scars, protects against free radicals, moisturizes and balances the skin, absorbs easily in your skin, minimizes fine lines and wrinkles, antimicrobial, evens skin tone, and many other mind blowing benefits. Grapeseed oil also cures the skin internally by intake of a ½ tbsp. with every diet twice a week.

Grapeseed oil is packed with antioxidants (like vitamin A, vitamin C, and vitamin E), omega fatty acids (like linolenic acid, an essential component of the skin's barrier), and amino acids (the building blocks for building collagen).

o **Normal skin type**: Grapeseed oil can protect against sun damage and promote collagen repair.

Grapeseed oil contains powerful antioxidants, minerals, vitamins, and fatty acids that work together to fade dark spots and lighten scars. Studies show that it can help speed up the healing process and decrease the formation of keloid scars.

- **Oily skin type**: High in linoleic acid, known as omega-6 fatty acid, which fortifies the skin's barrier which helps to reduce water loss from the skin, and helps with acne.

- **Dry skin type:** Reduces redness. Linoleic acid is known to be anti-inflammatory, and treats inflamed and red skin associated with breakouts.

- **Combination skin type:** Hydrates and firms. Grapeseed oil contains vitamin E which reduces inflammation, has moisturizing fatty acids, which may help skin appear tighter and younger.

- **Sensitive skin type:** Grapeseed oil is rich in compounds, including beta-carotene, vitamins D, C, E, and polyphenols. These compounds are antioxidant making grapeseed oil a free radical scavenging and protection from environmental aggressors such as UV radiation or pollution.

In Summary:

Grape seed oil moisturizes, boosts collagen, lightens dark circles, fades scars, tightens skin, and prevents sun damage. These benefits make it a fantastic addition to the Juicy By Mon Cheri cuticle oils helping to achieve a naturally radiating beauty for life.

HOW USING VITAMIN E OIL BENEFITS DIFFERENT SKIN TYPES

An essential nutrient found naturally in some foods including nuts, seeds and green vegetables, it has been a popular ingredient in skincare product for years. Although all vitamins including A, C, D, E or K are very important for a healthy and clear skin, Vitamin E is basically an oil-soluble antioxidant. Among eight different types of vitamin E, tocopheryl acetate and tocopherol are commonly used in skincare products. It can fight against free radicals and protects your skin from damage. It also has moisturizing and healing properties that help to boost the barrier function of your skin. Vitamin E can also be used to cure the wound scares on your face if applied mixed with unboiled milk. A few studies have shown that using Vitamin E oil can protect your skin from sunburn. Applying vitamin E oil on a sunburned area will soothe the skin and reduce the redness.

- **Normal skin type:** Protects, moisturizes, fades the look of dark spots, softens skin, improves texture, fights free radicals and calms the skin.

- **Oily skin type:** Vitamin E oil is not ideal for your skin type. It has the potential to clog your pores.

- **Dry skin type:** Helps provide moisture and allows the skin to retain water.

- **Combination skin type:** Vitamin E is a fat-soluble vitamin, which means that the skin not only readily absorbs it but holds it for longer than it may hold a water-soluble moisturizer.

- **Sensitive skin type:** Soothes and provides a protective barrier.

In Summary:

It protects, moisturizes, helps minimize signs of aging, softens skin, fades the look of dark spots, improves skin texture, soothes skin redness, acts as an antioxidant and strengthens skin. Vitamin E oil, adds lots of value to the Juicy by Mon Cheri oil's products helping you achieve naturally radiating and beautiful skin for life.

I have personally experienced the benefits using black seed oil, olive oil, grapeseed oil and vitamin E oil discussed in this book These oils are also included in the Juicy By Mon Cheri cuticle and body oils products available for purchase. Black seed oil has help me soothe and heal my nipples during pregnancy. I 've used black seed oil to heal myself , friends and family's open wombs for fast healing and so much more. Olive oil and grapeseed oil is used regularly on my scalp and body as a daily moisturizer. Vitamin E oil is used on new and old scars from surgeries or accidents to aid with skin tone evening. I often give my friends and family the gift of blackseed oil when in the hospital or when ill to aid in their healing process.

In summary, determining your skin type, as normal, oily, dry, combination or sensitive which may change from time to time depending on environmental factors will help you choose optimal oils and usage for your skin. Using black seed oil on your skin will aid in, healing, maintaining and improving your skin. Using Olive oil will moisturizes and fights bacteria on your skin . The Use of grapeseed oil will moisturize, boosts collagen and prevent sun damage. And Vitamin E oil will improve skin texture, fade dark spots while moisturizing and more. These oils are all conveniently included in Juicy By Mon Cheri oil products offering the most effective all-natural oil products for cuticle and skincare; to swiftly heal damaged cuticle and recover healthy nail growth, to promote even-toned skin from inflammation and early-ageing, and to achieve a naturally radiating beauty for life.

AUTHOR BIO

Mon Cheri Davenport

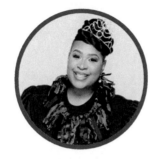

A Computer Engineer, Author, Ceramic artist, and self-proclaimed black seed engineer, Mon Cheri Davenport stands out for her passion and dedication to providing solutions to skin issues to her clients with outstanding results where other products have failed. Hailing from Cleveland, Ohio, Mon Cheri is a Computer and Communication Engineer by profession with over 20 years in the engineering industry. She holds a Bachelor of Science in Computer Engineering with a minor in Ceramic Art and M.S Bio-Medical Engineering.

Founder and CEO of Juicy By Mon Cheri, the company offers the most effective all-natural oil products for cuticle and skincare; to swiftly heal damaged cuticles and recover healthy nail growth, to promote even-toned skin from inflammation and early aging, and to achieve a naturally radiating beauty for life.

With more than 22 years of experience as a black seed oil enthusiast, Mon Cheri leverages her educational background and expertise to offer strategic and tactical insights, ultimately providing the best solutions to benefit her clients. Keen to share her knowledge and wisdom with others, Mon Cheri is the author of *"Healing Your Skin Through Natural Carrier Oils,"* an e-book with great insights into skincare management.

When she is not busy finding creative ways to solve skin care problems using black seed oils, Mon Cheri enjoys working out, listening to audiobooks and business podcasts, traveling, and being an art enthusiast.